Cut Your Health Care Costs Now!

By

Brandi Funk, FNP

About the Author

Brandi Funk is a board certified family nurse practitioner and health care advocate. Brandi graduated from Azusa Pacific University with a bachelor's degree in nursing in 1993 and a post master's degree as a family nurse practitioner in 2006. She has spent the last 15 years in her role as nurse researcher, clinician, and practitioner caring for and educating patients in hospital, retail health, and private practice settings.

Her most recent research on helping consumers cut their health care costs was inspired by watching her own family and patients, along with the rest of the nation, struggle to find affordable health care.

Brandi lives in southern California with her husband David and two boys, Jacob and Jarod.

Table of Contents

Introduction

The Cost of Healthcare is out of Control!

You don't need me to tell you. It's a national crisis. The cost of healthcare is painfully high with no end in sight. It's bad enough you work like a dog with little chance of getting that raise, you can't even afford to get sick! If you're like me, you watch the news, read the headlines and pray relief is coming soon. Relief through a national health care plan that will reign in costs and make health care affordable through competition and accountability in the health insurance market. A plan that will end discrimination against pregnant women and Americans with pre-existing conditions.

BUT...*You're going to have to wait until 2014!*

The $938 billion, 2,309 page health care Reconciliation bill signed into law March 23, 2010 requires 'fixes' in the Senate. This means the bill will be pulled apart, debated, and passed measure by measure. In addition, by the rules of reconciliation, each measure has to serve the purpose of cutting the federal budget. Looking at the size of the bill this could take a long time!

We will have to wait for the Senate to finalize the details and most changes will not take effect until 2014, but at this time, under The Reconciliation Act of 2010:

- 12-16 million people will remain uninsured.
- Illegal immigrants will not be eligible for assistance.
- In 2014, all Americans will be required to buy insurance from their employer, the government, or on their own or face fines. Penalty fees include:
  1. $95 or 1% of income, whichever is greater, in 2014.
  2. $695 or 2.5% of income, whichever is greater, in 2016. Family limit is $2,085. Low income, Native Americans & those with certain religious beliefs will be exempt.
- Americans may be forced to buy insurance they find too expensive or do not want.
- Government tax credits will help people who cannot afford to pay health insurance premiums. The aid will be available on a sliding scale to families with lower incomes, about $88,000 for a family of four.
- Insurers would be prohibited from rejecting applicants based on health status, but not until 2014.
- Later in 2010, insurers would not be able to exclude coverage for **specific** medical problems for **children** with pre-existing conditions, or set lifetime insurance coverage limits for children and adults.
- Insurers could still reject some children outright for coverage in the private insurance market until 2014.
- Annual limits on insurance coverage would be banned in 2014.

- People with a medical condition that has left them uninsurable may be able to enroll in a new federally subsidized insurance program that will be established within 90 days of the bill's passing.
- Unmarried adults can stay on their parent's insurance coverage until they turn 26, if they are not offered health coverage through their employer.
- Early retirees, 55 years and older and not eligible for Medicare, could get 80% of their medical claims over $15,000 (up to $90,000) reimbursed through the government reinsurance program until 1/1/2014.
- Over $400 billion will be taken from Medicare, including Medicare Advantage plans.
- In 2010, Medicare beneficiaries who reach the "donut hole" in the program's drug plan will receive $250. In 2011, the costs of drugs in the donut hole will be reduced by 50%. Eventually, the donut hole will be eliminated.
- Starting in 2010, preventive care for Medicare recipients will be free of co-payments or deductibles.
- Insurers will have to report how much they spend on medical care versus administrative costs and premium increases will be monitored by tighter government review.
- Small businesses with less than 25 employees and average wages less than $50,000 could qualify for a tax credit of up to 35 percent of the cost of their premiums.
- There will be an excise tax on certain medical devices.
- There will be a tax on cosmetic surgery and similar services.

Americans Are Suffering

"About half the families who file for bankruptcy do so at least in part because of health care debt."

– Harvard University, Joint Centers for Housing Studies

Americans are paying more out of pocket for healthcare and insurance. Even those with health insurance cannot afford care. Rising health care costs are keeping people from getting needed health care, bankrupting families, and endangering health.

Does this ring true for you & your family?

- Do you chip away at the credit card bills while deciding which prescription to refill?
- Are you struggling to find and/or pay for health insurance & costs?
- Are you feeling like there's no hope for getting the help you need NOW?

How this Book Can Help

Chances are if you live in America, if you are reading this book, you are in great need of finding help with the costs of healthcare now. I'm not going to tell you I have all the answers that are going to take your financial burdens away BUT I am excited to tell you that there's HOPE and HELP available!

This book does not claim to be the most exhaustive reference of healthcare saving options but instead, in my opinion, contains the most USEFUL information for you to use RIGHT NOW to save BIG on your healthcare costs!

I know you're struggling and I want to help.

I want to empower YOU to take back some control.

I've provided the "doors" for YOU to open!

Goodbye Google

You don't have to spend another minute searching aimlessly on the internet for help (you have better things to do!). I've done all the leg work for you, researching the healthcare industry and interviewing experts, to give you only the best insider tips and resources available so you can stop stressing and SAVE MONEY!

Isn't this GREAT news?

While some of these tips may not be new to you, many of them will be, showing you EXACTLY what to do and where to go to get help. I'll reveal insider "secrets" the healthcare industry doesn't tell or want you to know including:

- How to get the best health insurance for you and your family.
- How to prevent becoming "uninsurable" by insurance companies.
- How to get and keep health insurance with a chronic or serious illness.
- How to get medical care without health insurance.
- Where to get help with maternity care costs when it's excluded from your insurance plan.

- The right way to appeal an insurance claim denial that will increase your chance of winning by 80-90%.
- How to get the most out of your Medicare coverage.
- How to get a Medicare supplement with a pre-existing illness for the same price as healthy people.
- How to get your prescription drug costs lowered or FREE.
- How to negotiate your medical bills for up to half the "retail" price.
- How to save hundreds on your dental bills.

And much more!

So, are you ready to start learning how to save now?

Then, let's get started!

Chapter One

Buy the Best Health Insurance you can Afford

(And Read the Fine Print)

I understand that 14,000 Americans lose their health insurance coverage everyday **BUT** the truth is:

The best way to save money on your healthcare costs and protect yourself financially is to get health insurance. When you are *really sick,* health insurance is better than no insurance at all.

If you can afford it, a health plan that will cover your inpatient AND outpatient hospital expenses at best is better than no coverage at all.

Having health insurance will not only save you money on your out of pocket medical expenses, such as doctor visits, health tests, emergency care, and prescription costs, it can prevent bankruptcy and foreclosure on your home if you are hospitalized with a serious injury, need surgery, or are diagnosed with a life threatening or chronic illness.

One man that comes to mind, I met on the street a few months ago. He had recently lost his job with health insurance and a back surgery left him homeless with two very small children to care for.

You may be saying, "But I can't afford to buy health insurance."

This may or may not be true but YOU MUST EXPLORE ALL OF YOUR OPTIONS to try to find the most affordable insurance plan that will meet some if not all of your healthcare needs because:

Even if you find all you can afford is a catastrophic or high deductible health plan that covers your medical expenses in the event of a serious accident or illness, it can protect you financially from bankruptcy and foreclosure.

Health Plans 101

As you may already know, there are several different types of insurance plans you can buy privately or through an employer:

- HMO (health maintenance organization)
- PPO (preferred provider organization)
- EPO (exclusive provider organization)
- POS (point of service)
- Major Medical or Catastrophic

Make Sure You Know How Your Plan Works

If you've tried to read the insurance costs and benefits summary, you know the insurance companies do not make it easy to understand what we're buying. They list benefits and costs for in-network, out-of-network, physician co-pays, specialist co-pays, hospital inpatient and outpatient coverage, plan deductibles, drug pricing for formulary, non-formulary, retail, mail order, brand and generic drugs, etc.

It can be nearly impossible to know *what* **you're signing up for!**

Understanding your health insurance plan can save you a lot of money in the long run so it's very important to know exactly what you're buying.

When choosing a plan, the most important thing for you to know is that typically:

- HMOs cost you less each month with limited access to physicians and specialists (think referral).

- PPOs cost, on average, double the HMO monthly fee, allowing you more access to physicians and specialists of your choice, whether they are in or out of the plans network.

- EPOs are similar to PPOs with the exception that they usually do not cover out of network physicians and specialists.

- POSs are a combination of an HMO a PPO. They cost much less than PPOs and EPOs. They don't have a network and a referral by a primary care doctor is needed to see a specialist.

- Major Medical or catastrophic plans have low monthly premiums with high deductibles ($1,000-$10,000) you have to pay *before* they cover routine and major medical costs. Most plans do not cover maternity costs.

For a more detailed but simplified explanation of health insurance options in your state, I recommend *The Consumer Guide for Getting and Keeping Health Insurance* at http://www.healthinsuranceinfo.net..

Important Things to Consider Before Choosing a Plan:

According to a recent *Consumer Reports* investigation, there are many "junk" health plans with loopholes, limits, and exclusions that can be financially devastating. Before you sign, put your plan to the test with these important questions.

- ✓ Premiums – How much will it cost you each month. How much will they increase each year? What's the grace period for payments?

✓ Coverage/benefits - What is the **lifetime MAXIMUM?** Does it include vision & dental? Will it cover your chronic illness?

✓ Does the plan pay for preventive health care?

✓ Does it cover inpatient AND outpatient hospital care? **DO NOT** sign up if it covers "hospital only." The majority of surgeries, dialysis & cancer treatment are done outpatient.

✓ Access to **YOUR** doctors, hospitals, and other providers (you can usually check online). How do you access them? Do you need a referral?

✓ Access to after hours and emergency care.

✓ Out-of-pocket costs (coinsurance, co-pays, and deductibles) **Be sure there's an out of pocket maximum (NEVER sign up without one) and that your costs are 100% covered after your deductible is met.**

✓ Prescription drug coverage – What is the **maximum annual drug coverage** and which drugs are covered. Check to see if your monthly Rx meds are on their formulary.

✓ **Exclusions** and limitations, including **PREGNANCY** (This section is very important so READ THE FINE PRINT!).

✓ How are claims paid? Will you have to submit a claim after paying out of pocket? What is the time limit for claim submission?

Self-Funded vs. Fully Funded Health Insurance Plans

The Employee Retirement Income Security Act of 1974 (ERISA) governs health insurance plans provided by private employers nationwide. ERISA law requires that employer health plans comply with the federal HIPAA law when it comes to covering certain illnesses *and pregnancy.* It does NOT apply to government and church employee plans.

Employee health plans are either self-funded or fully funded

Under a **fully funded insurance plan**, the employee buys commercial health insurance from an *insurance company.*

The insurance company assumes the risk for payment of claims and **is regulated under state law. It is subjected to rules about mandated benefits, network adequacy, prompt payment of claims, etc.**

Under a **self-funded insurance plan,** the employer pays claims out of its own funds and **is NOT regulated under state law or subjected to rules about mandated benefits, network adequacy, prompt payment of claims, etc.**

What this means for <u>YOU</u>

- State insurance departments have no authority to investigate complaints that involve self-funded plans.
- Certain medical conditions and related treatments and supplies may NOT be covered.
- State laws requiring mandated (required by law) health benefits and coverage do not apply.
- Self-funded insurance claim denials are NOT eligible for state external review.

Private Insurance plans are always fully funded

Private insurance plans are fully funded so they are regulated under state law and must follow rules about mandated benefits, network adequacy, and prompt payment of claims.

Checklists for Diagnosing Your Coverage

- ➢ Use this checklist at <u>http://www.kff.org/consumerguide/05-checklist.cfm</u> to better understand the scope of your insurance coverage as a way of steering clear of potential issues.

➤ *Consumer Reports* has created a standardized form with more questions to help you clarify your plan's cost and coverage at http://www.consumerreports.org/cro/resources/streaming /PDFs/cost_coverage.pdf.

You <u>must</u> review your health plan for changes in coverage anytime:

- Marital status changes

- Number of dependents change

- You, your spouse or dependent's residence changes

- You, your spouse or dependent terminate or begin employment

"How do I choose the best plan?"

Getting the "Best": It's All About Quality

In our culture, quality is often associated with higher costs. Yet, in medicine, this is not usually the case. Research studies have proven time and again that in healthcare, there is no link between quality and spending. This means insurance premiums are a poor gauge of healthcare quality.

In fact, healthcare organizations have shown that they can produce high quality healthcare at lower costs.

As the consumer, you expect to receive high quality care no matter the cost including:

- Getting preventive care.
- Timely access to care.
- Seeing a specialist when needed.
- Obtaining care, tests or (appropriate) treatment believed necessary.

I don't want to just give you a phonebook of all of the plans that "hang out a shingle" but the right information to help you buy a plan that *truly* protects you at a price you can afford.

America's Best Plans

The National Committee for Quality Assurance, a private, non-profit organization dedicated to improving health care quality, and U.S. News & World Report have put together a detailed ranking of over 600 commercial, Medicare, and Medicaid HMO and POS plans in America. Rankings are based on member satisfaction and success in preventing and treating illness compared with other commercial plans. You can also search by state, region and insurance plan name.

Find Top-Rated Plans at:

America's Best Health Plans 2009-10

http://health.usnews.com/health-plans

Health Plan Report Cards

Go to http://reportcard.ncqa.org for a report card on how well your insurance plan performs.

Compare two plans side by side, looking at:

- **Doctors and Hospitals:** Are the doctors and hospitals you prefer included in the plan's network? Are those doctors and hospitals near your home or work?

- **Benefits and Services:** How well does the plan cover you and your family's health needs — the ones you can anticipate, as well as potential emergencies? *Does it offer prenatal and maternity care?* Is your prescription medicine covered?

- **Value:** How much will you need to pay out of your own pocket in the form of **co-payments** and **deductibles?** What is your monthly premium?

State Department of Insurance

Your state insurance department is another resource for evaluating insurance company performance. You can look online for information on each company doing business in your state.

The two most important pieces of information you want to look for are:

- Number and type of complaints filed against them.
- Medical loss ratios (a fancy term for the amount of money they spend, or "lose" as they see it, on healthcare).

The average ratio is between 70 to 80 percent. More money spent on healthcare = less executive salaries. Some states have minimum requirements for medical loss ratios.

FYI, the higher their medical loss ratio, the lower their stock falls, leaving their investors very unhappy.

YOU want to be their priority NOT their investors!

Visit http://www.consumeraction.gov/insurance.shtml for your State Department of Insurance

Visit http://reportcard.ncqa.org for more information on how to choose a health plan.

For **health insurance options available in each state,** go to the Georgetown University Health Policy Institute's website at http://www.healthinsuranceinfo.net or the National Association of Health Underwriters website at http://www.nahu.org.

One More Thing You Should Know...Gender Rating

In 38 states, private insurers can charge women who purchase individual insurance 2%-48% more on average for the same coverage than men, a practice called gender rating. Federal law bans employers of more than 15 employees from this discriminatory practice but only 12 states make it illegal.

If you are a woman, you should know if this practice is legal in your state.

Gender Rating is Illegal or Limited in:

- New York
- Minnesota
- New Hampshire
- Montana
- North Dakota
- New Mexico

Washington

Vermont

Maine

Massachusetts

Oregon

New Jersey

Chapter Two

Health Plans: The Good, the Bad and the Ugly

Finding a Plan

So you know the different types of insurance plans available and what to look for.

Now, where do you get health insurance?

1. Your Employer

The best way to ensure that you are covered, regardless of whether you are sick, is through your employer. With these plans, insurances cannot refuse to cover you due to a pre-existing condition BUT they can make you wait:

- 12 months if you received medical advice, diagnosis, care, or treatment within the past 6 months. If it has been longer than 6 months, the prior condition cannot be subject to a pre-existing condition exclusion.

- Up to 18 months if you enroll late so **enroll during your first open enrollment opportunity**.

BONUS; the money you spend on your insurance premiums through your employer is taken out of your paycheck **first,** so it is **NOT included in your taxable income**.

Also, if you lose your job, get your work hours reduced, or divorce, you may be eligible to continue your health coverage under the Consolidated Omnibus Budget Reconciliation Act (COBRA) for up to 18 months (29 months if you're disabled). Your spouse and dependents can get coverage for up to 36 months.

I will talk more about COBRA a little later.

Do Not Pass Go Until You Read This!

The majority of employer health plans are **self-funded,** which means **certain medical conditions and related treatments and supplies may NOT be covered under your employer plan** and **state** health insurance mandates DO NOT apply.

For example, coverage for in vitro fertilization is a required mandate in the state of Georgia and Hawaii BUT if your employer offers a **self-funded** insurance plan these laws do not apply. This means they would not have to cover this or any other medical treatments under their plan. In addition, self-funded plan denials are NOT eligible for state external reviews (see chapter 4).

However, these plans must comply with federal Employee Retirement Income Security Act (ERISA) laws, which require they comply with the HIPAA law and federal mandates when it comes to covering certain illnesses *and pregnancy*.

See page 116 for more information on state health care mandates.

YOU NEED TO KNOW...

ERISA laws DO NOT APPLY to government and church employee plans.

Contact your Employer's human resources department to find out if they offer a self-funded (vs. **fully funded**) plan and *pay close attention to plan limitations and exclusions*. See **page 24** for more information on Self-Funded vs. Fully Funded health plans.

Are you a federal employee?

2. Federal Employees Retirement System (FERS) - Federal employees, retirees and their survivors are fortunate to have the largest selection of health, dental and vision plans in the U.S.

Visit the **Federal Employees Health Benefits Program** webpage at http://www.opm.gov/insure/health/planinfo/index.asp for a detailed list of plans with links to provider directories in each state.

NEW! The American Recovery and Reinvestment Act (ARRA) of 2009 allows former federal employees who were involuntarily terminated between September 1, 2008 and May 31, 2010 to request health insurance premium assistance for temporary continuation of coverage (TCC) under the Federal Employees Health Benefits (FEHB) Program. This means your former agency may contribute 65 percent of your TCC premiums for up to 15 months.

Are you (or about to be) unemployed?

3. Change your employer group plan to an individual plan

Before your employer-based coverage expires, ask if you can convert your current group health plan to an individual policy. Many states require this "conversion right" to be included in group health insurance contracts. A few states allow the insurer to choose whether to have a conversion option or a continuation option in its health insurance. Individuals eligible for a conversion policy are on a guaranteed issue basis (coverage cannot be denied) and cannot be subjected to pre-existing condition exclusion periods.

Conversion policies can be very expensive with limited benefits. Some states have rules establishing minimum benefits that conversion policies must cover and maximum rates that can be charged.

Visit www.statehealthfacts.org to find out if your state offers conversion policies.

4. Consider COBRA

The Consolidated Omnibus Budget Reconciliation Act (COBRA) gives workers who lose their health benefits the right to choose to continue group health benefits provided by the plan under certain circumstances. Unfortunately, some church and small employer plans may not be required to offer COBRA benefits.

You may qualify to continue your health insurance under the following circumstances:

- If you voluntarily or involuntarily lose your job; other than "gross misconduct"

- If you have reduced hours of work
- If you become entitled to Medicare
- If you get a divorce or legal separation
- If you are the spouse of a covered employee who dies
- If you lose status as a "dependent child" under plan rules

Employees can receive coverage under COBRA for up to 18 months (29 months if you are disabled within the first 60 days of COBRA coverage) and their spouse and dependents can get coverage for up to 36 months. Visit http://www.cms.gov for details.

I hate to break it to you but if you extend COBRA coverage to 29 months due to disability, your insurance carrier **can increase your premium up to 150 % of the cost of coverage** during the 11-month disability extension.

Do You Want the Good News or the Bad News First?

The bad news is that continuing coverage under COBRA is expensive, up to 102% of the cost of your employer plan, and many simply cannot afford to pay the monthly premiums on their own.

The good news is that under The American Recovery and

Reinvestment Act of 2009 (ARRA) you could be eligible to pay only 35 percent of your COBRA premiums while the remaining 65 percent is reimbursed to the provider through a tax credit. To qualify, you must have lost employment between September 1, 2008 and May 31, 2010.

The premium reduction **applies to periods of health coverage that began on or after February 17, 2009** and lasts up to 15 months.

Keep in mind…This subsidy phases out for individuals whose modified adjusted gross income exceeds $125,000, or $250,000 for those filing joint returns. Taxpayers with modified adjusted gross income exceeding $145,000, or $290,000 for those filing jointly, do not qualify for the subsidy.

For more information call 866-444-3272 or visit http://www.dol.gov/ebsa/cobra.html.

Very Important!

Do everything you can to pay your COBRA payments ON TIME, even if you do not receive a bill (remember, they don't care if you default).

By law, insurance companies must give you a 30-day grace period for payment of premiums BUT I've heard of cancellations before the grace period.

The take home message here is that your COBRA coverage **CAN BE CANCELLED IF YOU ARE LATE OR DELINQUENT ON JUST ONE PAYMENT** so pay on time. I highly recommend you arrange for an *automated* monthly payment through your former employer if possible.

Do <u>NOT</u> Skip this Part!

What I'm about to tell you may mean the difference between you having health insurance and you becoming UNINSURABLE.

You have **63 days** to switch your health plan to COBRA, a private or government plan, your spouse's plan, or a plan with a new employer (unless they have a 90 day waiting period) or **you risk being unable to get insurance anytime in the near future**.

If you have a serious medical condition or chronic illness, chances are very high you will be "uninsurable'" by private insurance companies who usually exclude coverage for 'pre-existing' conditions.

COBRA may be the only coverage you can get until you can switch to another employer-based plan.

Under HIPAA, insurers cannot deny you **full** coverage as long as you switch from one plan to the next within 63 days (more in some states) and your earlier coverage lasted for at least a year.

Visit http://www.dol.gov/ebsa/faqs/faq_consumer_cobra.html or call 1.866.275.7922 to learn more about COBRA coverage.

5. Find an Insurance Broker

Disclaimer: "Insurance agents have a financial incentive to sell insurance coverage, even if that coverage may not be the best financial product for the consumer."

With that in mind, when choosing an agent, ask for a referral from friends and family and check to see if they are licensed in your state.

But no worries, by the end of this book you will be ready to face the insurance broker!

If you opt out of your employer's plan, are unemployed or self employed, you can find private health insurance coverage through a reputable insurance broker from the Independent Insurance Agents & Brokers of America at www.iiaba.net or through www.einsurance.com.

Be Aware these plans often cost more, with higher co-pays and deductibles and fewer benefits. The key is to shop around and give yourself plenty of time to look over and choose the right plan.

Unlike employer health plans that have to accept everyone at the same price, in most states, private health plans are underwritten based on your age, weight, smoking status and past and present health history.

Plan Deductibles

To keep costs down, you may want to consider a **higher deductible plan** if and **ONLY** if:

- You are healthy.
- You can afford the deductible and want to save on monthly premiums.
- You don't need any prescription drugs.
- You don't have any pre-existing or chronic illnesses.

- You can afford high out of pocket expenses.
- You don't plan on getting pregnant at least for the next 12 months.
- The plan covers inpatient AND outpatient hospital care.

Here's where it gets ugly…

Maternity Care: It May NOT be Included in Your Plan

DID YOU KNOW? Most **individual** insurance plans in **America** <u>DO NOT</u> cover the cost of maternity, leaving 1 out of 3 pregnant women under insured or uninsured. In fact, only 12% of the 3,500 individual private insurance policies sold in the U.S. cover comprehensive maternity care.

Here's what a woman recently wrote to the *Colorado Independent News:*

"Just three days ago I found myself stunned, angry, and discriminated against when I learned that my individual health insurance plan (nor any individual plan) doesn't cover maternity care. I am a consultant, newly married and we're planning on having children. Even though I can enroll in his group health plan, I shouldn't have to. I am outraged, but not surprised, that insurance companies can get away with this (not to mention the exorbitant price of having a baby)." –Chris

"What about HIPAA?"

Well, are you ready for this…under the Health Insurance Portability and Accountability Act (HIPAA), health care plans cannot consider pregnancy a pre-existing condition, even if the woman did not have previous coverage, BUT this applies mainly to employer or **GROUP** insurance plans.

Unfortunately, there are **no federal laws requiring private insurance companies to provide maternity coverage** and many insurance companies have found loopholes within HIPAA laws.

State Mandated Maternity Coverage

At this time, only 5 states**: Massachusetts, Montana, New Jersey, Oregon,** and **Washington** have mandated laws requiring all insurance companies in their state to cover maternity costs. Individual insurance providers in New Jersey and Washington are allowed to offer "bare bones" health plans that are exempt from the mandate. Other states have limited coverage mandates.

Another reason to get and keep your employer's group plan when at all possible. A **self-insured** employer that offers **group** health benefits, if it includes maternity coverage, cannot exclude a new employee's pregnancy under a pre-existing condition clause.

Health Care Reform and Maternity Coverage: Under the new health care legislation, beginning in 2014, all insurance plans must provide maternity care coverage.

Until then, if you are left out in the cold...

I recently heard about a young couple in Arizona who didn't read the fine print and received a bill for $30,000 after a normal childbirth delivery (5x the cash or fair market price). If this has happened to you, STOP here, go to chapter four and read how to negotiate your bill.

The Bottom Line...

Know Your Rights!

A great resource for learning more about federal and state protections can be found at: www.healthinsuranceinfo.net/guides_map.htm.

This website has a separate guide for each state.

Make Sure You're Covered

If you choose a private health plan, especially one with a high deductible, be sure it includes MATERNITY COVERAGE or consider adding what they call a MATERNITY RIDER to your plan upfront to cover birthing expenses not covered by your plan. DO NOT WAIT because some insurance companies will not let you add this later! For example, Blue Cross Blue Shield of Tennessee will not let a woman add the benefit after she initially purchases a policy unless she submits an official "notification of change in status" and gets married.

Call your insurance broker or visit **Maternity Health Insurance.Org** at www.maternity-health-insurance.org for quotes online.

EXCEPTION: If you are sure you will not need maternity coverage, you can save money here. In this case, check your plan to ensure you are NOT paying additional for this benefit. Sometimes it is automatically added so it's important to check.

BUYERS BEWARE!

I have to be honest with you about these RIDER plans. Depending on your state, they can be very hard to get with long waiting periods, a list of disqualifying terms and conditions and offer very poor maternity coverage, $2,500 on average.

Other Options (NO assistance should NOT be an option):

- Buy a more comprehensive medical plan that includes maternity care.
- Call the U.S. Uninsured Help Line (800) 234-1317.
- ONLY if you cannot get insurance - consider a **discount** medical plan.

Be aware! There are many scams out there. The only **discount plan** I can recommend is **Best Benefits**, a reputable company with a high consumer satisfaction rating and backing by the Consumer Health Alliance, which sets standards for discount healthcare companies to operate with integrity, fairness and accountability. They offer a 30-day money back guarantee.

You can search for providers and hospitals online. I was pleased to find a large number of OB GYN physicians in their network. Read pages 88-89 for more information about discount cards.

- **Negotiate a cash price** with your physician or midwife and hospital *upfront, before* your prenatal care begins or risk paying up to 10 times the amount you would pay with insurance! You can also negotiate your bill after you have received medical care. (See chapter four on how to negotiate pricing).

- Ask your obstetrician and hospital for your insurance's contracted price for your prenatal care and delivery, even if you're not insured for maternity care.

- Consider **disability insurance**. Most moms do not know they can get disability insurance during pregnancy if they're unable to work (this includes severe morning sickness & doctor ordered bed rest). The terms will vary from state to state. Go to www. disability.gov for information in your state.

If your state does not offer disability insurance, ask your employer if they offer it for a fee or group rate. If you are already covered by disability insurance through your job, maternity disability insurance should be included. You can also purchase DI on your own through many insurance companies, ideally BEFORE pregnancy or as early as possible. For quotes and information, visit www.2insure4less.com.

- Consider state funded maternity care programs. Find eligibility and applications for your state at: www.medicaidapplication.org/default.asp.

- Use a state funded health center near you at http://findahealthcenter.hrsa.gov. These centers can also help you with applying and getting government financial assistance.

Alabama: Hope for improved Maternity Coverage

Alabama is leading the way to improve maternity care. As of January 1, 2010, they will offer a "revamped" maternity care program to substantially improve quality, services and access. Visit http://findahealthcenter.hrsa.gov to read more.

Did you lose your job to goods & labor moving overseas?

6. Trade Adjustment Assistance Reform Act

If you have recently lost your job because of trade policy (increased jobs and imports moving overseas), you may qualify for government help that allows you to pay 65% of the cost of your health insurance for a year or longer.

Visit the **Health Coverage Tax Credit** (HCTC) website at www.irs.gov/individuals/index.html or call the customer contact center at 866-628-HCTC.

Are you unemployed and "uninsurable?"

7. State Guaranteed Issue Plans

If you have exhausted all of your options of finding a health plan, it may be worth looking into what is called a "guaranteed issue" plan. Under HIPAA law, insurance companies in each state must sell health plans to anyone in need.

Unfortunately, HIPAA does not limit how much premiums can be charged so these plans are not ideal. They may only cover the bare minimum with catastrophic coverage in exchange for **high premiums and deductibles**. Often there are low maximum payment caps on prescription drugs, which can be useless if you have a chronic medical condition. Visit www.statehealthfacts.org or call (202) 347-5270 for information in your state.

8. State High Risk Pools

Another last option, high risk pools are special insurance plans subsidized by the government to cover those who are "medically uninsurable," who've been denied coverage for a pre-existing illness or who've been offered plans that are too restrictive and extremely expensive. Plans are purchased from state approved private insurance companies who are monitored by the state for compliance.

With High Risk Pools:

- You must have exhausted all other resources to be eligible.
- You may be required to show two proofs of denial letters from insurers.
- Premiums and out of pocket expenses for these plans are much higher than individual insurance, with caps placed by the government.
- Despite the high costs, there are usually waiting lists of 6-12 months.

In October 2009, Blue Shield of California was "ousted" from the state's high risk medical pool because its premiums were too high.

Do I hear cheering?

State high risk pools are **available in 35 states**

Visit www.ncsl.org or call 202-624-5400 for a list of all state health programs that cover the uninsured, including high risk pools.

Are you self-employed?

If you are self-employed, you can buy private health insurance through an insurance broker (see page 39) or through the National Association for the Self-Employed. They do not offer a policy in every state but they may be worth looking into.

Learn more at www.nase.org and check with your tax advisor to see if your premiums are tax deductible.

9. Memberships:

You can buy health insurance through memberships such as:

- City Chamber of Commerce
- Professional Organizations
- Trade Associations
- Alumni Clubs
- Labor Unions (i.e. The Union Labor Life Insurance Company http://ullico.com offers hospital expense protection, life, accidental death & dismemberment, dental and vision plans)
- AARP (American Association of Retired Persons) www.aarphealthcare.com has several plans available for ages 50-64.

Are you an early retiree under age 65?

While Americans are working longer, most retire before they are eligible for Medicare benefits. It used to be employers paid employees' health care benefits until Medicare kicked in.

Today, this is less and less the case. Whether you are forced out of your job or choose to retire early, finding a health plan to bridge the gap can be difficult and costly.

This explains why most early retirees are just "hanging in there" without any coverage until Medicare begins.

Do not let this happen to YOU.

Consult with an insurance broker

Health insurance can be expensive in your 60's BUT insurance companies want your business when you turn 65, hoping you will buy a supplemental or Advantage policy, so odds are good they will give you a reasonable quote.

See page 50 "Memberships" for other health insurance options including:

- AARP (American Association of Retired Persons) at

www.aarphealthcare.com. They have several plans available for ages 50-64.

10. Federal Pension Benefits Guaranty Corporation

If you are a retiree aged 55 or older, your former employer no longer provides your pension, and your pension benefit is paid by the federal **Pension Benefits Guaranty Corporation**, you can receive help with 65 percent of the cost of health insurance until you are eligible for Medicare.

Learn more about this option at www.irs.gov/individuals/index.htm or call 866-628-HCTC.

Have children?

11. The Children's Health Insurance Program Reauthorization Act of 2009 (CHIP)

Children in America should not go without health care coverage. Unfortunately, more than 5.1 million jobs have been lost in the recession, leaving more children without health insurance coverage than ever. If you have recently lost your job and/or your employer based health insurance and your annual income has dropped below an average of $44,000 (for a family of 4) your children may qualify for government help.

Consider 70 percent of uninsured children nationally are eligible but not enrolled for public insurance programs. According to the federal government, this is mostly because too many parents do not know that help is available and how to apply.

In a big effort to change this, President Obama passed the *Children's Health Insurance Program Reauthorization Act of 2009 (CHIP)*, designed to help families who do not qualify for Medicaid but cannot afford private health insurance.

To help enroll as many eligible kids as possible, they have increased income eligibility levels and simplified the application process.

The new federal law includes fiscal incentives for states to enroll eligible low-income children in Medicaid. Also, dental services are a required benefit and legislation allows federally qualified community health centers to contract with private dental practices to provide care.

For more information and applications in your state, visit **Insure Kids Now** at http://www.insurekidsnow.gov/state/index.html.

For Older Children - Some states have defined who is eligible for dependent coverage under fully insured group and individual health insurance policies. Under the new healthcare bill, beginning in September 2010, dependent children will be allowed to stay on their parent's insurance until age 26, unless they are offered insurance through their employer. Visit http://www.statehealthfacts.org for information in your state.

For Children with Disabilities visit Social Security Disability Insurance (SSDI) benefits at http://www.ssa.gov.

See page 91 for additional resources.

One Size Does Not Fit All

I have presented many different health plan options, depending on your current situation. One plan for everyone may not be best. After examining your options, I encourage you to consider the plan that is best for you *and* each member of your family.

See if your children qualify for CHIP or SSDI and if you and your spouse or partner qualify for other types of coverage before you buy a family plan or go without insurance altogether. Doing this could cut your health care costs significantly.

Learn more about your health care options by visiting **The Foundation for Health Coverage Education**® website at http://www.coverageforall.org.

There you will find:

The Health Care Coverage Eligibility Quiz - Answer five questions to help determine for which programs you and your family qualify.

The Health Care Options Matrix™ Guide - Download and print your state's FREE reference guide to all the public and private health care options. Includes a reference list of phone numbers and websites.

The U.S. Uninsured Helpline - Call 800.234.1317 and speak to a live operator any time-24 hours a day, 7 days a week.

Health Insurance Companies from A to Z

Visit www.ahip.org for a complete list of insurance companies.

Chapter Three

The Medicare Maze

Are you 65 years or older, disabled or have ESRD?

12. Medicare

Medicare is the government healthcare program for Americans 65 years and older, some disabled, and those with end stage renal disease (ESRD). U.S. citizens and legal aliens of 5 years or more are eligible for Medicare if they or their spouse worked for at least 10 years in Medicare-covered employment. Be sure to sign up for Medicare about three months before you reach age 65.

There are 4 parts of Medicare coverage:

- Part A – Inpatient hospital coverage. **Usually** no monthly premium (if you or your spouse paid Medicare taxes while working) but a $1,100 deductible for inpatient hospital care < 60 days and $155 yearly deductible for regular medical care. For more information on Part A, call Social Security at 1-877-772-5772 or visit www.socialsecurity.gov.

- Part B – Outpatient medical coverage. Includes a monthly premium ($96 - $110 in 2010). The monthly premium amount is available in the "Medicare & You" handbook produced by the U.S. Centers for Medicare and Medicaid (CMS) and on the Medicare website at www.medicare.gov.
- Part C – Medicare Advantage plans that combine A, B, D.
- Part D – Prescription drug insurance. You pay an additional monthly premium and a $310 initial deductible for 2010.

Do Not Enroll Late or it will Cost You!

Important: You do not have to be retired to enroll in Medicare. **Initial enrollment for Medicare Part B begins 3 months before you turn 65 until 3 months after**. If you do not enroll during this time, you will have to wait for the general enrollment period, between January 1st and March 31st each year. If you are still working, contact the Social Security office to find out when the best time is for you to enroll in Part B because you will have to start paying monthly premiums. If you receive Social Security retirement benefits, you will automatically be enrolled in part A the month you turn 65.

Except in special cases, the cost of Medicare Part B will go up **10%** **for each full 12-month period** that you could have had Medicare

Part B but did not take it. **You will have to pay this penalty as long as you have Medicare Part B.** This can really add up!

If you are a federal employee covered by federal employee health benefits plan (FEHB) and continue to work past Medicare eligibility **you will not have to pay the 10% penalty increase.**

Initial enrollment for Medicare part D begins 3 months before your turn 65 until 3 months after (3 months after your 25th month of cash disability payments if under a disability plan). If you do not sign up when you are first eligible, you may pay a penalty. If you did not join when you were first eligible, the next opportunity to join will be from November 15th to December 31st each year.

To find out if you are eligible for Medicare and when you can enroll, go to www.medicare.gov/MedicareEligibility/home.asp or call the Social Security Administration at 800- 772-1213.

Medicare and Federal Employees

If you are a retired federal employee, learn how the Federal Employee Health Benefits (FEHB) Plan and Medicare work together. Read *Medicare: Basic Information and Considerations for Federal Employees* at www.myfederalretirement.com and the **U.S. Office of**

Personnel Management website at:

www.opm.gov/insure/health/medicare/index.asp.

Medicare for Disabilities and ESRD

If you are already getting Social Security retirement, disability benefits, or railroad retirement checks, you will be contacted a few months before you become eligible for Medicare and given the information you need.

You should contact Social Security about applying for Medicare if:

- You are a disabled widow or widower between age 50 and age 65, but have not applied for disability benefits because you are already getting another kind of Social Security benefit;
- You are a government employee and became disabled before age 65;
- You, your spouse or your dependent child has permanent kidney failure;
- You had Medicare medical insurance in the past but dropped the coverage; or
- You turned down Medicare medical insurance when you became entitled to hospital insurance (Part A).

For Children with Disabilities visit Social Security Disability Insurance (SSDI) benefits at http://www.ssa.gov/pubs/10026.pdf.

See page 91 for additional resources.

Medicare Help

The State Health Insurance Assistance Program, or SHIP, is a national program that offers one-on-one counseling and assistance to people with Medicare and their families.

If you want to know more about the SHIP program in your state, or you want to contact a SHIP counselor in your area, visit Shiptalk at www.shiptalk.org.

For more in- depth information on Medicare, I recommend reading the *"Medicare & You"* handbook produced by the U.S. Centers for Medicare and Medicaid (CMS) available on the Medicare website at www.medicare.gov.

Medigap Insurance vs. Advantage Plans

Understanding Medicare insurance supplement options and which one is best for you could **save you a lot of money and frustration!**

Because Medicare does not cover *all* medical expenses, people who do not have other medical insurance can choose to buy additional coverage, either a Medigap policy **or** a Medicare Advantage Plan.

Medigap Plans (Medicare Supplement Insurance)

A Medigap policy is health insurance sold by private insurance companies to fill the "gaps" in original Medicare Part A and B.

With these plans, you continue to use traditional Medicare as your primary insurance and the Medigap as your secondary insurance to help cover the cost of what Medicare does not cover.

Open enrollment for Medigap plans begins the first day of the month you are 65 or older and enrolled in Medicare Part B and ends 6 months after. During this time, Medigap insurance companies cannot refuse to sell you any plan if offers. **If you do not enroll during this time, insurance companies do not have to sell you a policy and can charge you more.**

As of 2006, Medigap policies cannot include prescription drug coverage because Medicare Part D provides it. So, if you need prescription drug coverage, you will have to buy a Medicare prescription drug plan (Part D) offered by private insurance companies approved by Medicare. The average premium in 2010 is $32 a month and includes a $310 initial deductible.

Enroll in Part D when you are eligible for Part B or you may pay a monthly penalty.

Find the **Medicare Prescription Drug Plan Finder** at http://www.medicare.gov.

Medigap Coverage for People Under 65

Unfortunately, not all states are required by law to sell Medigap policies to people under age 65 with disabilities, leaving many without this option.

For more information and a list of states that do offer Medigap policies for people under age 65, read *Medigap Policies For People Under Age 65 With A Disability or End-Stage Renal Disease (ESRD)* at www.medicare.gov/medigap/under65.asp.

Medigap Coverage with Pre-existing Conditions

While Medigap insurance companies cannot make you wait for your coverage to start, they can refuse to cover pre-existing health conditions for up to six months, if you had the condition during the last 6 months before Medigap coverage starts. Your original Medicare will still cover you during this time.

However, not all Medigap insurance companies can make you wait so do your homework. If they do make you wait, when you buy a policy during your Medigap initial open enrollment period, the insurance company must shorten the waiting period for pre-existing conditions by the amount of creditable coverage you've had. For example, if you had Medicare part A and B for 4 months prior to your Medigap policy starts, the insurance company must use the 4 months as credible coverage and shorten the waiting period to 2 months instead of 6 months.

If you had Medicare for more than six months before you turned 65 years old, you will not have a pre-existing condition waiting period because Medicare counts as creditable coverage.

For more information read *Medigap Coverage of Pre-existing Conditions* at www.medicare.gov/medigap/prex.asp.

Guaranteed Issue Rights

READ CAREFULLY...

Normally, insurance companies can use medical underwriting to accept or deny your application and how much to charge you for a Medigap policy BUT if you enroll in a Medigap plan during your *initial* open enrollment period, you are guaranteed coverage under what is called "Guaranteed Issue Rights." During this specified time, **you can buy any plan you want, even with a pre-existing illness, for the same price as people with good health. Also, if you lose certain kinds of coverage within 63 days, insurance companies cannot use a pre-existing condition waiting period.**

Remember, you will have to have had **prior credible health coverage with no more than a 63-day gap** before you apply for Medigap and your enrollment begins when you are eligible for Medicare part B until 6 months after, so do not be late!

Read more in Section 3 of *Choosing a Medigap Policy: A Guide To Health Insurance For People With Medicare* at www.medicare.gov/Publications/Pubs/pdf/02110.pdf.

NOTE: If your medical coverage ends before you turn 65, you can send in your application for a Medigap policy before your Medigap open enrollment period starts so there are no breaks in coverage.

Each insurance company decides which Medigap policies it wants to sell so shop around and compare plans.

For more information and help choosing a Medigap plan, call 1-800 633-4227 or download *Choosing a Medigap Policy: A Guide To Health Insurance For People With Medicare* at http://www.medicare.gov/medigap . This guide describes how other health insurance plans supplement Medicare and offers some shopping tips for people interested in those plans.

The Truth about Advantage Plans

Advantage Plans are health insurance sold by private insurance companies. Although you are still covered under Medicare, you sign your Medicare benefits over to an HMO or PPO in exchange for them to "manage" your healthcare.

All Beneficiaries Pay

Insurance companies that sell Advantage plans collect an extra 12%-19% for each policy from the government. *That's an average of $1,100 more per beneficiary per year than traditional Medicare, almost $44 billion between 2004 and 2008!*

Excessive overpayments to these plans are a burden to **ALL** Medicare beneficiaries, including those who are not enrolled in them.

Is there an Advantage?

Despite what some call, "extremely aggressive and deceptive marketing practices," many seniors are reported to be happy with their Medicare Advantage plan. Advantage plans are attractive because of initial low premiums and out of pocket expenses. In addition, some plans offer other benefits not covered by traditional Medicare or Medigap, including dental, prescription drug, and wellness programs. Finally, Advantage plans usually cover pre-existing conditions, which Medigap is not always required to do.

Initial enrollment for Medicare Advantage plans begins when you become eligible for Medicare Part B until 3 months after. Annual open enrollment is from January 1st to March 31st each year. You can also make changes to your existing Advantage plan or switch back to Original Medicare during this time.

Wait! Before you sign, there are a few things to consider. If you are in relatively good health, these plans may be better than traditional Medicare with a Medigap supplement BUT advocates warn they have heard seniors complain about not knowing what they were signing up for including:

- Restricted choice of doctors and hospitals.
- High deductibles and co-pays when sick.
- High increases in premiums.
- Voided certain retiree benefits.
- Inability to get a Medigap supplement when switching back to original Medicare.

Something to Think About

Insurance companies are increasingly denying claims, which is a big problem if you have an illness.

Attorney and healthcare advocate Jennifer Jaff, founder of **Advocacy for Patients** www.advocacyforpatients.org, warns that it is very difficult to win an appeal of denial of coverage under Advantage plans.

Jaff says, "I haven't lost one appeal to traditional Medicare," something everyone with a serious or chronic illness should bear in mind when considering their options. The bottom line is that you have to read the fine print to know exactly what you are buying.

Check out the best Medicare plans at http://health.usnews.com and **Medicare plan report cards** at http://reportcard.ncqa.org.

Important Changes in 2010

The Medicare market is changing. In 2010, government subsidies to Advantage plans will decrease slightly but there will still be a $3.60 per month increase in Medicare monthly premiums.

Due to the decrease in subsidies, Medicare says Advantage plan premiums will increase by 25% in 2010 with the number of available plans dropping by more than 40%.

Some seniors are already seeing their plans disappear and dramatic increases in premiums.

In 2010, we will also see a decrease in Medicare part D "stand alone" plans.

The Prescription Drug Gap (Donut Hole)

The Medicare prescription drug gap or so called "Donut Hole" requires Medicare Part D enrollees to pay 100% of the total drug costs after their covered medications exceeds the initial coverage limit of $2,830 (in 2010), before exceeding the catastrophic coverage limit of $4,550 (in 2010).

Some plans have lower drug cost coverage of say $1,800, so if you have high prescription drug costs you may want to consider which plans offer additional coverage until you spend $4,550 out-of-pocket.

This gap in coverage is generally above $2,830 in total **retail** (not what you pay personally) drug cost, until you spend $4,550 out-of-pocket.

Even so, with these plans, you may pay less for your prescription drugs than you would without this coverage.

According to the Kaiser Family Foundation, "There is growing evidence that some enrollees who reach the gap forgo needed medications when faced with the full cost of their prescriptions."

Visit http://www.q1medicare.com for more information about Gap coverage and just about everything related to Medicare, including an online donut hole calculator, part D checklist, Rx Savings Finder and enrollment tips.

Can you believe? Some plans **charge up to three times** as much for generic drugs in the gap than the initial coverage. In this case, you want to be sure to use an Rx discount card and search the Rx Savings Finder so you do not end up paying full price. See chapter five for more information.

NEW! As part of the new healthcare reform bill, Medicare Part D recipients who have reached the donut hole will receive a $250 check from the government in 2010. Checks will start going out in June.

Closing the Gap:

- Consider keeping your employer or former employer's drug plan.
- See if you qualify for low income assistance at www.kff.org/medicare/upload/7327-05.pdf.
- Switch to generics or lower costs drugs – See chapter five.
- Apply for extra help at www.socialsecurity.gov or call 1-800-772-1213.
- Search for help from charitable programs at www.benefitscheckup.org.
- Keep using your Medicare drug plan card even while in the gap so you get discounted prices.
- Purchase a stand-alone prescription drug plan.

Medicare Part D Stand Alone Plans

Traditional Medicare does not cover outpatient prescription drugs and Medigap plans sold after 2006 do not cover prescription drugs so you will have to enroll in a part D "stand alone" plan if you do not have prescription drug coverage through a Medicare Advantage plan. Part D stand-alone plans are purchased from insurance companies approved by Medicare and cost about $32 a month.

Initial enrollment for Medicare part D begins 3 months before you turn 65 until 3 months after (3 months after your 25th month of cash disability payments if under a disability plan). If you do not sign up when you are first eligible, you may pay a penalty and will have to wait for the next open enrollment from November 15th to December 31st each year to join.

Visit www.medicare.gov to find and compare drug plans.

Compare drug pricing within different plans at **DestinationRx** http://plancompare.destinationrx.com and the RxSavings Finder at www.q1medicare.com.

Review Your Medicare Plan Every Year

Doing this could save you a bundle! Each year Medicare sends recipients an "Annual Notice of Change" describing changes in premiums, deductibles, copayments and coverage. You have from November 1st to December 31st to make any changes, including changing insurance plans and carriers.

I recommend shopping around during this time to be sure you are getting the best deal.

Compare Medicare health plans at www.medicare.gov or www.q1medicare.com (review list of best plans and report cards; see links on pg. 69).

Look for changes in:

- Premium hikes – Can you afford them?
- Prescription drug co-pay hikes - More plans are changing from fixed co-pays to a percentage of the cost of the drugs. It could mean an increase or decrease in prices.
- Are your prescription drugs still covered? Many are added and dropped every year.
- Decreased coverage – i.e. dental care.

Note: Know what circumstances give you Guaranteed Issue Rights during this time if you want to make changes in your health plan.

For example, if your Medicare Advantage insurance company leaves Medicare or moves out of your area, you have a Guaranteed Issue Right. This would be a good opportunity to get insurance without any underwriting, which is especially important if you have a pre-existing illness.

Is Your Income Low?

If you cannot afford to pay your Medicare premiums and other medical costs, you may be able to get help from your state, which may have programs for people entitled to Medicare with low income.

These programs may pay some or all of Medicare's premiums, deductibles and coinsurance.

"To qualify, you must have Part A, a limited income, and in most states, your resources, such as bank accounts, stocks and bonds, must not be more than $4,000 for a single person or $6,000 for a couple."

For **more information**, read publication *Get Help with Your Medicare Costs* (Publication No. CMS-10126) from Medicare at http://www.medicare.gov/publications/pubs/pdf/10126.pdf.

13. Medicaid

Medicaid is government paid health insurance that helps many people who cannot afford medical care pay for some or all of their medical bills.

Medicaid also helps cover some costs not covered by Medicare.

You must qualify to receive benefits. There are many different programs to help adults and children get medical care.

Visit http://www.cms.hhs.gov/apps/contacts to learn about the Medicaid program in your state, including eligibility.

Chapter Four

Medical Bills: How to Play the Game to Win

Get the Best Price

Recently, I fell in love with one those expensive, designer purses at our local mall. After looking at the price tag, I knew I could not afford it.

I *really* wanted this purse! But, I needed a *better* price so I could buy it.

So what did I do?

I went home, got on the computer, and began my quest.

After about 30 minutes, I was able to find my purse, along with several other less expensive knock-offs, for 20% less than the mall price!

The day *AND* my pocketbook were saved!

While you may not be into designer purses, I'll bet you comparison shop too. Most of us do. Not just for expensive things, but for everyday things like an oil change, tires, shoes, eyeglasses, groceries laundry soap, and even toilet paper.

Doesn't it feel good to know you're getting a good deal?

But how do you know you are?

YOU COMPARE PRICES!

You wouldn't dream of buying a new car without knowing the fair market value, let alone drive it home and wait for the bill!

Why is it different when it comes to healthcare?

Why can't we shop around for the best deal?

I'm here to tell you...YOU CAN!

We've sat back for too long not knowing (or caring) what that test, procedure, treatment or surgery is going to cost until we get the bill. Usually, it's not until we see in black and white what we're going to have to pay out of our own pocket that we feel differently about the price.

We've seen a shift in this way of thinking in the cosmetic and elective plastic surgery industry where it's cash only driven.

Within this market, men and women are very motivated to shop for the best price. Don't believe me? Google™ "best price for breast augmentation" and see how many websites come up – 7,080,000! You will find prices clearly listed and very competitive. In fact, prices for breast augmentation have remained steady over the last 10 years and the industry is BOOMING!

You've <u>Got</u> to Shop Around

This is not only important if you are uninsured. Thanks to rising deductibles and co-insurance (percentage you must pay), there are a growing number of people with insurance who are paying more of their health care out of pocket.

If you want to save big on your healthcare cost, you have to know how much it *should* cost, according to fair market value and where to get the best price *before* the service is provided. The problem with doing this in the past was that prices were kept "Top Secret" by medical establishments and insurance companies, giving them an unfair advantage.

Today, thanks to new fair healthcare pricing laws and websites, we are starting to see a more level playing field and the game is changing in our favor.

Think you *always* get a better price through your health insurance?

Think again.

Would you be surprised if I told you that sometimes you can get a *better* price paying cash than going through your insurance company?

It's time you knew the truth.

Healthcare Transparency: The "Secret" is out

The federal government's push to increase people's awareness of their health care spending goes hand-in-hand with getting hospitals, physicians and health insurance companies to share more price information. State legislatures argue, "More people have a reason to know what they spend on health care, due in part to the increasing popularity of high-deductible health insurance." As a result, some states have passed 'fair pricing' laws.

California: The Hospital Fair Pricing Act

In California, patients who do not have health insurance have the right to receive discounted hospital services.

A landmark law, effective January 1, 2007, makes it illegal for hospitals to charge uninsured patients more than what Medicare or Medicaid would pay for hospital care.

This means they pay *the same rate* for the same care as government programs.

Well, they are *supposed* to anyway. California compliance audits show this law has not been successfully implemented in hospitals.

Recently, auditors found that less than two-thirds of all hospitals surveyed had the required notices posted in both the admissions area and the emergency room. In addition, forty-three percent of hospitals surveyed were unwilling or unable to give their financial assistance policies to surveyors on request, as required by law.

Web-based Health Care Price Disclosure Guides

HealthcareBlueBook.Com (www.healthcarebluebook.com)

To find fair market value prices for surgery, hospital stays, doctor visits, medical tests and dental work, I highly recommend Healthcare Blue Book. Just enter your zip code and the procedure or test and they will give you a fair estimate of what it should cost based on solid data for FREE. You can then use this price to shop around and negotiate a fair price.

Remember the couple in Arizona who recently received a bill for $30,000 after having their baby? According to Healthcare Blue Book, the "fair market" cash price for their new bundle of joy is about $6,000, a $24,000 difference! It's unfortunate they did not know this because they could have used this information to negotiate a fair price upfront with their doctor and hospital.

They are now negotiating down their medical debt with the hospital, which is harder to do.

According to Kathleen Stoll, Health Policy Director for Families USA, pregnancy and childbirth are perfect to price ahead of time, giving many families peace of mind and an opportunity to plan.

NewChoiceHealth.Com (www.newchoicehealth.com)

With NewChoiceHealth, Inc consumers can lookup medical facilities and compare costs for common procedures such as MRIs, EKG, Mammograms, and more. Enter your city and state to shop locally or Nationwide from over 20,000 medical facilities for over 400 of the most commonly performed medical procedures.

Because it only offers pricing for medical procedures, New Choice Health is not as comprehensive as Healthcare Blue Book.

PriceDoc.Com (www.pricedoc.com)

PriceDoc™ connects you to affordable, quality doctors and dentists in your area. Enter your zip code and the procedure or specialty and you will be connected with physicians in your area along with their profile. You can then make a direct online request for cash prices. Some providers list the cash price for you to 'click and reserve.' You can also "name your price" for the procedure you need. Once you enter an amount that you can afford, they will let you know when a local provider has accepted your price.

The Chapman Consulting Group (800)906-8085 (www.hospitalbillreview.com/medicare.php) has information for every procedure by every hospital so if you want to know what Medicare would reimburse you for a hospital visit or physician, they have the information and can help you understand your bill.

State Sponsored Health Care Price Disclosure Websites

Sixteen state hospital associations have cost and comparison shopping websites for common inpatient procedures.

Other states have their own systems.

Visit www.healthcarebluebook.com for a list of state websites.

Visit:
www.ncsl.org/IssuesResearch/Health/DisclosureofHealthandHospitalCharges/tabid/14512/Default.aspx for proposed legislation and laws in each state.

Scroll down to view:

- ✓ **"Web-based Provider and Hospital Price Disclosure Plans"**
- ✓ **"Private Insurance Company Price Disclosure Websites**
- ✓ **Table 1: State Legislation Relating to Health Care Price Disclosure.**

The Centers for Medicare and Medicaid Services (CMS) http://www.cms.hhs.gov/HealthCareConInit has posted the cost and Medicare payments for over 60 procedures at ambulatory surgery centers and over 40 procedures performed in inpatient hospitals but this information is limited and not very helpful in my opinion. For more comprehensive information on Medicare costs and payments, I recommend **The Chapman Consulting Group.**

Success Stories

Healthcare Blue Book CEO Dr. Jeffrey Rice has many success stories from people who have used the website to lower their medical costs. He recently told me about a woman with Medicare looking for a better price for a medical test. "She called and said, 'your prices are wrong. It says it should cost about $500 but the price I was given (locally) was $2,500.' I suggested she check with other providers in her area. She called another provider with the $500 quote from Healthcare Blue Book. They told her they could not do it for that price but that the provider across the street could. When she called them, they told her they could do the test for $300." This was a significant savings for her, having a 20% Medicare co-pay. She ended up paying $60 out-of-pocket instead of $500

Is your insurance company giving you the best price?

During our conversation, Dr. Rice brought up an interesting point, "Sometimes paying cash up front is better. One woman paid 20% *less* than she would have through her insurance company by paying cash instead," crediting Healthcare Blue Book for giving her the "fair market" cash price before her appointment. He said he knew specifically of insurance companies that consistently charge their members more than the fair market price for services.

I say it's because they can get away with it and urge you to play it smarter by knowing what your medical needs *should* cost upfront.

Negotiate Your Price *First*

If you are paying cash or you know your procedure will be out-of-network, call the hospital billing department to negotiate *before* the procedure. It is much easier, and your chances of getting a good deal are much higher if you talk to your physician *before* rather than *after* you receive care. **This is especially important if you need expensive testing, medical treatment, surgery or maternity care.** Once you have dealt with the hospital, try talking to the surgeon, anesthesiologist and other specialists involved.

Remember…Quite often you will find that the hospital will be contracted (in network) with your insurance company and the physician will not be and vice versa or that neither are contracted. If this is the case, always **ask for your insurance's contracted price for your care. Ask for the contracted price for all insurance policy exclusions** (pregnancy, surgery, cancer, etc.)

Recently, my mother needed a heart procedure in an outpatient hospital. The test was not covered and the hospital was not contracted with her insurance company so they quoted her the $1,200 "retail" price. At the time, she had not heard about fair pricing websites, such as Healthcare Blue Book, so she had no idea what the test *should* cost.

As she was discussing the price with the woman scheduling her test, the woman said, "Let me call your insurance company and see if I can get you the 'contracted' price." Sure enough, she was given the negotiated insurance price of $500 and paid even less than that when it was all said and done!

Although the hospital was not contracted, she still received her insurance's discounted rate.

Most hospitals are not going to tell you this so you have to ASK.

Financial Help for Serious and Chronic Illnesses

Quite often, people ask me how they can save or afford care for a serious or chronic illness such as cancer, multiple sclerosis, autism, etc. so I have provided some additional resources for special circumstances.

For online pricing for cancer treatment, Healthcare Blue Book is a great resource. Type "cancer" into the search box and you will receive pricing for various types of cancer treatment.

Insurance Options

Please read **chapter one** for information on health insurance options and **chapter five** for financial assistance for prescription drugs.

Survivorship A-Z has a **Health Plan Evaluator** www.survivorshipatoz.org/hpe.php for cancer, HIV, and other health conditions that helps you sort through your priorities and determine which of several health insurance plans is best for you.

Also, I found many oncologists and specialists are in network with the Best Benefits discount plan. See page 89.

Discount Health Cards

Many people choose to buy a discount card to complement their health insurance program, filling in gaps, such as prescription drug coverage, hospital, emergency, physician, chiropractic, hearing, dental or vision care. They can be a great option for both the underinsured and uninsured to lower out of pocket expenses.

Discount cards allow you to buy healthcare products and services from providers at a discount similar to those you would receive through insurance plans. Discount cards are gaining in popularity. Many of the country's Fortune 500 companies now offer discount cards to their employees as part of their benefits packages. Signing up for a card is easy. Complete an application and pay a low monthly fee.

Scam Alert!

Unfortunately, not all discount card plans are reputable and you could fall victim to a scam if you do not ask the right questions upfront. I advise reading, *"A Consumer's Guide to Choosing the Best Card and Company"* from The Consumer Health Alliance before choosing any discount card at: www.cbplan.com/Images/pdfs/CHA-Consumer-Guide.pdf.

Best Benefits Discount Plan

After a lot of research and investigation, I am only able to put my "stamp of approval" on one discount plan, **Best Benefits**.

This plan is managed by Discount Development Services LLC, a division of Coverdell & Company, Inc., a founding member of the Consumer Health Alliance, the trade association of providers of discount health plans. This means you can be assured of the quality of the Best Benefits plans and the company's ethical practices.

Best Benefits discount plan (www.healthcaresavingslink.com) **is NOT health insurance** or substitute for insurance but a discount plan that finds healthcare providers who are willing to provide discounts. Backed by the Consumer Health Alliance, the Best Benefits plan is a nationally recognized leader in the non-insured discount health care marketplace.

Founded in 1995, **Best Benefits** is the largest provider and manager of reduced fee health care plans in the country with over six million members across the United States.

Participating providers are screened by a team of professionals and must pass strict criteria prior to joining the network.

- Choose from three different plans ranging in price from $8 to $18 a month for a family membership.

- Search for providers in pharmacy, chiropractic, dental, vision, hearing, physicians, specialties, and hospitals, urgent care, marriage and family counselors, massage therapists, cosmetic surgery and more through **Beechstreet Health Corporation** (www.beechstreet.com), one of the nation's leading preferred provider organizations.

I did a local search for providers in various medical specialties (OB GYN, Pediatrics, family practice, oncology, marriage and family counseling) and was impressed to find hundreds of results for physicians, including many of my own.

Government and Private Assistance

State Sponsored Programs (http://www.needymeds.org/state_programs.taf) – Search for programs offered in your state.

HealthWell Foundation (http://www.healthwellfoundation.org/) - Provides financial assistance to eligible individuals to cover coinsurance, copayments, healthcare premiums, and deductibles for certain diseases and treatments.

PSI (Patient Services Incorporated) (http://www.uneedpsi.org) Provides assistance to those with certain chronic illnesses or conditions with the cost of health insurance premiums associated with COBRA, state high risk pools, open enrollment, Guaranteed Issue policies, HIPAA conversion policies, and prescriptions co-payments associated with private insurance and Medicare Parts B and D.

State Directory (www.patientadvocate.org/report.php) of information for financial relief for a broad range of needs including housing, utilities, food, transportation to medical treatment, and children's resources.

Patient Access Network (PAN) Foundation (www.panfoundation.org) - Helps the underinsured access the health care they desperately need to continue living a relatively normal and productive lifestyle. Every day Patient Access Network helps thousands of underinsured patients afford the copayments for their cancer or chronic disease medications.

The Chronic Disease Fund (www.cdfund.org) - Supports patients with more than a dozen different diseases, including many types of cancer (breast, colorectal, and lung cancer, and multiple myeloma), rheumatoid arthritis, multiple sclerosis, asthma, and macular degeneration, to name a few.

Low Cost to Free Health Centers

(http://findahealthcenter.hrsa.gov)

The Hill-Burton Program - Sponsored by the federal government, provides funds to hospitals for the treatments for people who are low income and would not be able to afford expensive, long-term treatments. Ask your local hospital about the program or call 1-800-638-0742 to find a participating hospital in your area.

National Cancer Institute's Cancer Information Service

(http://cis.nci.nih.gov) 1-800-4-CANCER (1-800-422-6237).

Clinical Trials (www.clinicaltrials.gov) – a registry of federally and privately supported clinical trials conducted in the United States and around the world. Recommended reading: *Should I Enter a Clinical Trial? A Patient Reference Guide for Adults with a Serious or Life-Threatening Illness* at www.ahip.org.

Susan G. Komen Breast Cancer Foundation www.komen.org.

American Cancer Society (www.cancer.org).

Cystic Fibrosis Patient Assistance Program (www.cfpaf.org).

Women's Health (www.womenshealth.gov) - The federal government's source for women's health information.

Cancer Care (www.cancercare.org) - Provides grants to help cancer patients cover the cost of cancer treatment expenses, but they also provide financial aid to help patients pay for the additional childcare or home care expenses incurred during therapy. Call 1-800-813-HOPE for a financial assistance application.

Co-Pay Relief www.copays.org (through the Patient Advocate Foundation) -Assists insured patients with certain cancer diagnoses.

Transplant Fund (transplantfund.org) – Helps raise money and administer funds for medical expenses of patients and living donors not covered by insurance.

American Kidney Fund (www.kidneyfund.org) - Helps more than 75,000 kidney patients in the United States with health insurance premiums, Medicare Part D expenses, and other treatment-related expenses that insurance will not cover.

Health Insurance Assistance Service (HIAS/ACS) - Assists cancer patients who have lost or are in danger of losing their health care coverage, along with identifying policy solutions to help others in similar situations. 800-ACS-2345.

First Hand Foundation (www.cerner.com/firsthand) - Helps with medication, surgeries, medical equipment and travel related to an ill child's care. Additionally, the foundation implores doctors, hospitals and equipment providers to discount their services below listed prices.

Helping Hand - Financial Assistance for Autism. (www.nationalautismassociation.org/helpinghand.php)

Autism Cares Foundation (http://autismcaresfoundation.org) is a Pennsylvania-based nonprofit organization that assists directly to families and caregivers of individuals with autism. The foundation's support is intended to enhance services provided by other agencies as well as provide additional support that may not be otherwise available.

The Autism Treatment Center of America (www.autismtreatmentcenter.org) Financial assistance for families and caring professionals wanting to help their children by attending the *Son-Rise Program*® training courses. Call 413-229-2100 and speak to a family counselor.

The State Medicaid Title XIX MR/DD Waiver Program (http://www.wid.org/publications/directory-of-publicly-funded-pas-programs) Under the Waiver program, a parent's income is waived when determining children's eligibility for Medicaid. Medicaid Title XIX provides health care coverage for individuals with Mental Retardation and/or Developmental Disabilities **(including autism & Aspergers)**. Reimburses for services to instruct, intervene, support and assists individuals who have mental retardation and/or related conditions to achieve the highest level of independence and self-sufficiency possible in their lives.

Directory of State Title V CSHCN Programs (http://mchb.hrsa.gov/programs/) Every state and the District of Columbia has a Title V Program **for Children with Special Health Care Needs** (CSHCN) which provides funds to states to develop and operate public health care programs for certain children with special health care needs.

Friends of Man (www.friendsofman.org) – Provides Food, Clothing,

Medicine, Prostheses, Wheelchairs, Eyeglasses, Dentures, Medical Equipment, Daycare, Training and Education, Hearing Aids, and more.

Airline Flights for Treatment & Evaluation

Organizations that provide free air transportation for stable patients to distant treatment facilities:

Corporate Angel Network (http://www.corpangelnetwork.org)

Air Charity Network (http://aircharitynetwork.org)

Mercy Medical Airlift (http://www.mercymedical.org)

National Patient Travel Center (http://www.patienttravel.org)

Lowering Your Medical Bills

DID YOU KNOW?

An uninsured or underinsured person who goes to a hospital is charged 3 to 5 times more than an insured person would pay for exactly the same care. **There are two lists of prices: one for the insured and one for the uninsured.**

Do not let them to take advantage of you!

Ask for a Discount

Remember, when it comes to lowering your medical bill, *you're in charge*. Most medical bills are negotiable. The majority of people that ask for a discount from their provider or hospital –the right way- get it! In fact, most hospitals expect you to ask and are ready to give you a substantial discount if you know what you are doing.

You have to ask and may have to insist!

It is a well-kept secret; many hospitals in the United States are *required* to provide some free or low cost care, or what's called "charity care," to uninsured or low-income people who cannot otherwise afford to pay their bills.

Check with the hospital billing or financial office. Be clear and confident stating, "These bills are extremely high. Would you consider lowering them?" Ask if the hospital will "write off," "forgive," or cancel some of your bill.

At the very least, ask if you can get the same price as insurance companies. Find out what the cost would be for Medicare and from websites like HealthCareBluebook.com and negotiate from there.

If they agree, get it in writing. If they don't, ask to speak to the chief financial officer and ask for a reduction to the hospital's actual cost plus 25%. Add that you are willing to pay cash up front if the price is affordable. If it's not, ask if you can make payments without accruing interest.

If they still will not work with you, call in a pro. See page 102 for a list of bill **negotiation services and advocates who can negotiate your bill on your behalf.**

Advocacy groups like the Chapman Consulting Group www.hospitalbillreview.com can determine how much you should reasonably pay and coach you on what to say to hospitals and providers.

Finally, if you have bills from doctor's offices, call them right away and see if you can get a discount and/or make payments without interest. Many providers are willing to work with patients and reduce their fees. Turn down any offers to pay with one of their credit cards, even if it is 0% interest. Once you pay with a credit card, you lose your power to negotiate.

If it is an emergency and you are stuck with an out-of-network doctor, call your insurance company to help you resolve the issue.

Check the Laws in Your State

Community Catalyst's Free Care Compendium
(www.communitycatalyst.org/projects/hap/free_care) summarizes the free care laws and regulations in each of the fifty states.

Remember…If you are genuinely in need for charity and are receiving multiple bills and threats of legal action, they cannot pressure you or demand payment.

I Always **Ask**

I have a high deductible (and two teenage boys) so paying $100 dollars or more out of pocket after each physician visit to meet my deductible can be a hardship. Recently, I received a bill from our family orthopedist for $185. I called their billing department, explained that this was a financial hardship and asked if they could lower the amount. After waiting on hold for a few minutes, they offered me a $25 discount and the option to pay them back in three installments, interest free. It was not as big of discount as I wanted but I was happy to have saved something.

I bet YOU can do better! Get help if you need to.

A word of caution: some medical providers may offer you a credit card or a loan to repay your bills. You should avoid these because they usually have high interest rates or penalties if you make a late payment.

Check Your Bill for Errors

Over 90% of medical bills have errors. Hospitals make $10 billion a year off intentional and unintentional billing errors. According to the New York Life Insurance Company, the average medical bill has $600 worth of errors. This not only comes out of your insurance company's pocket, it comes out of yours.

The first thing you want to do when you receive a bill is ask for an itemized copy of the charges.

Look for:

- **Double billing:** Check your bill for double charges for the same service, supplies or medications.
- **Tests that were not done:** Verify that all tests on your bill were performed.
- **Days in Hospital:** Be sure you are being charged for the correct number of days you were in the hospital.

- **Room Rate:** Hospitals have different rates for private, semi-private, two-person and four-person rooms. Make sure they match what you actually had.

- **Up-Coding:** A common practice where a less expensive item is charged as the more expensive one, i.e. generic vs. brand name drugs.

- **Check the equipment usage:** How many days of oxygen were used?

- **Keystroke Errors:** Check for extra or missing numbers.

- **Charges that say "Misc."** or other nonspecific descriptions.

Bill Negotiation Services

Organizations and companies that can help you understand and negotiate your bill:

- **Hospitalbillreview.com** (The Chapman Consulting Group) (http://www.hospitalbillreview.com) (800)906-8085

- **Billadvocates.com** (http://www.billadvocates.com)

- **Patientadvocate.org** (http://www.patientadvocate.org)

- **Healthproponent.com** (http://www.healthproponent.com)

- **Healthchampion.net** (http://www.healthchampion.net)

- **Healthcarebluebook.com**
  (http://www.healthcarebluebook.com)
- **Claims.org** (http://www.claims.org)
- **Smart Medical Consumer**
  (http://www.smartmedicalconsumer.com) will help you
  manage medical expenses, with break through features
  including automatic detection of medical billing mistakes.

Always **Submit a Claim for Reimbursement**

This past fall I paid out of pocket for me and my family to get a flu shot at a retail health clinic that was not contracted with my insurance. The provider printed out a claim form with my receipt for me to fill out and send in to my insurance company.

A few weeks later, I was quite happy to find a reimbursement check in the mail for $90 dollars.

Even if you are told or do not think your insurance company will cover a physician, test, procedure, etc., submit an insurance claim for reimbursement anyway. If it will save the insurance company money in the long run, they may go ahead and reimburse you.

Ask your provider to submit the claim for you or ask for a claim form with instructions and fill it out yourself. Ask them or your insurance company for help if you need it. Sure, it will take some extra time and effort on your part but it may be well worth it. What do you have to lose?

Give Yourself a (Tax) Break

Sign up for a Flexible Spending Account

Flexible spending accounts (FSA) are set up by employers as part of their benefits package. With an FSA, you reserve money from your paycheck, BEFORE taxes are withheld, to use to pay for your out-of-pocket health care and dependent care expenses.

You save money by paying *less* in taxes.

Let's say you make $2,000 per pay period, which means you pay taxes on $2,000 per pay period. If you put $20 per pay period in a FSA, you only pay taxes on $1,960. Use the FSA Calculator at www.fsafeds.com/fsafeds/fsa_calculator.asp to calculate your potential tax savings.

What's great about FSAs is that you can use the money to pay your co-pays, co-insurance, deductible, prescription and over-the-counter drugs, other medical expenses that your regular insurance does not pay for, such as vision, chiropractor dental, and child and adult daycare, tax free. See all **qualified medical expenses** at www.irs.gov.

You must have a high deductible health plan to participate, $1,200 for self and $2,400 for family in 2010.

What's not so great is that **you have to forfeit any unused money at the end of the year.**

Archer Medical Savings Account for Self Employed

If you are self-employed or work for a small company with less than 50 employees, you may qualify for an Archer Medical Savings Account through a bank or insurance company.

For More Information, visit: www.irs.gov/publications/p969/ar02.html#en_US_publink1000204 112 .

Health Savings Account

A health savings account (HSA) is similar to a FSA. They are used with high deductible health plans.

The major differences are:

- Balances are not forfeited at the end of the year.
- The account is not closed after employment is terminated.
- The account can be transferred to another HSA or Archer Savings account.
- Money can be spent on non-medical expenses (with penalty & taxes).

Read all about HSAs at www.treas.gov/offices/public-affairs/hsa/pdf/all-about-HSAs_072208.pdf.

Retail Healthcare Clinics

If you really want to keep your medical costs down, avoid the ER and urgent care, where you have little control over your costs, whenever possible.

Retail healthcare clinics like **MinuteClinic** and **Take Care**, located in pharmacies and other stores, are a growing trend in the U.S.

If you have ever been to a retail clinic, you can easily see why:

- No appointment needed.

- Convenient hours 7 days a week.
- Low cost (all services and costs are posted) outside the door.
- You can get treatment for whatever is ailing you in about 15 to 30 minutes.

Using a retail healthcare clinic can save you hundreds of dollars.

I used to work as a nurse practitioner for one of these clinics and I can't tell you how many patients I saw who commented about how much time and money they were saving versus going to the ER, urgent care and their physician.

One woman came to see me with a urinary tract infection. She told me that she had gone to the ER for the same problem 2 months ago and received a bill for $1,500. Her visit with me was just $62 (without insurance) AND she was in and out with her prescription within 45 minutes!

Did I mention their high patient satisfaction ratings?

Worried about the quality of care at a retail clinic?

A large study published in the Annals of Internal Medicine in late 2009 found "retail clinics offer quality service for a lot less than physician offices and urgent care centers."

For some services, retail clinics did slightly better than hospital emergency rooms.

Travel a lot? You can find a retail clinic throughout the U.S.

Visit **MinuteClinic** (www.minuteclinic.com) 866-389-2727 or **Take Care** (www.takecarehealth.com) 866-825-3227 for locations, services, costs and contracted insurances.

Find a Low Cost or Free Clinic

Federally funded health centers take care of you, even if you have no health insurance.

Health centers are in most cities and many rural areas. Go to http://findahealthcenter.hrsa.gov to find a low cost or free clinic near you.

Avoid Unnecessary Tests & Procedures

When my friend John was told his 75 year old, frail father needed a colonoscopy, he assumed it was because his doctor believed he *needed* one.

He was surprised, confused, and later angry when he learned there was no medical indication for his father to have the test.

He had agreed to the test and said that the bowel prep before the test left his father very weak, taking him days to recover.

He says it's hard to find peace with himself and the doctor who made the decision for his father to have the test adding, "I have regretted allowing them to do this test because I didn't speak up about whether he needed it or not."

It is a well known fact that unnecessary tests and procedures are driving up the cost of healthcare. A survey of Massachusetts doctors found 83 percent had ordered unnecessary tests, hospital admissions and referrals at a cost of $1.4 billion a year in that state alone. The cost is $700 billion nationwide. This not only comes out of your insurance's pocket but it comes out of yours as well.

Now, I know a lot of you believe that doctor always knows best but I urge you to question any tests, procedures, surgeries, referrals that you aren't absolutely convinced you need.

Ask your doctor these questions:

- Why do you (or a loved one) need the test?
- What is it going to show?

- What are the short and long-term effects?
- What if you don't get the test or procedure?
- Is there a less expensive test or procedure? (i.e. Ultrasound vs. CT scan).
- Is this going to change your treatment plan or help fix the problem?
- Is it covered under your insurance?
- How much will you pay out of pocket?

If the answers are not clear or convincing, do not agree to have the test or procedure done. Doing this could save you a lot of grief and potentially thousands in the long run.

Fight Back! The Right Way to Appeal a Denial

So your insurance plan has denied you coverage, what do you do?

Do not accept the insurance company's word as final.

The Department of Labor estimates that about 1 in 7 claims made under employer health plans that it oversees is initially denied.

This is a growing trend that is sure to affect all of us. Fortunately, we have a right to appeal these decisions. Unfortunately, only about **4% of denied claims are appealed.**

According to attorney and patient advocate Jennifer Jaff, founder of **Advocacy for Patients** (www.advocacyforpatients.org), if you want to dramatically increase your odds of winning an appeal:

1. **DO NOT listen to the insurance company when they tell you to call** to request an appeal over the phone.

2. **Make the request in writing**.

The denial letter may say, "If you want to appeal, give us a call." Then what's your appeal? They are just going to look at the same information that they have already looked at. What you need to do is gather your medical records and send them things that they haven't looked at before that illustrates how necessary your treatment is.

3. **Get medical records**.

It is not enough for your physician to write a letter to the insurance company on your behalf.

Ms. Jaff states, "If you write a letter that says that you need the treatment and are really sick without it, it won't work. Getting your medical records shows how you were doing before you used the particular, let's say it's a drug, and how after, it worked in your case.

That's the kind of evidence that you need. It needs to be in the medical records."

4. Appeal *before* treatment

Ms. Jaff adds, "The appeal before treatment is really critical because you can't get the treatment unless you win the appeal, or you can't get the insurance company to pay for the treatment unless you win the appeal. An appeal after treatment is all about money. The appeal before treatment is not about money, it's about your health.

5. Appeal before the deadline

Ms. Jaff warns, "If you blow the deadline on filing your appeal, you're done. I cannot stress enough the importance of meeting that deadline. People just kind of ignore that, and then they're surprised when the insurance company says we're not even going to let you appeal."

Appeal Letters: Write to Win

Ms. Jaff has provided **step-by-step instructions** at
http://advocacyforpatients.org/insurance_training_material.pdf

that includes appeal letter templates for writing an appeal that will dramatically improve your chances of winning.

For Medicare appeals, read "How to File an Appeal," on page 87 of the *"Medicare & You"* handbook produced by the U.S. Centers for Medicare and Medicaid (CMS) available on the Medicare website at www.medicare.gov.

More Appeal Letters & Forms

For more appeal letters and information, **Appealletters.com** (www.appeallettersonline.com) has:

- Over 1500 downloadable medical appeal letters

- How-to articles on denial management

- Downloadable forms and other information resources to help improve your denial management success

- Searchable database to find what you need quickly & easily

- Members-only discussion forum

- Knowledge-building online seminars & training tools and slideshows

- Audio conferences on a multitude of appeal topics

- State Resources with links to court cases, state statutes and other resources for every state

- Case studies reveal successful practices of other medical facilities

Get Help from your State: External Appeals

If you have a non-ERISA or non-employer, private insurance plan, you have a right to appeal any decision of denial by your insurance company through an independent external review organization, usually through your state department of insurance.

These reviews can be very beneficial as they are truly independent and unbiased and they can overrule insurance companies.

Go to www.kff.org/consumerguide/states.cfm for information on external appeals in your state.

Please note: with self-funded plans, plan denials are NOT eligible for state external review.

Get Help from an Advocate

Patient Advocate (www.patientadvocate.org) can assist you with your insurer, employer and/or creditor regarding insurance, job retention and/or debt crisis matters relative to your diagnosis of life threatening or debilitating diseases.

The Chapman Consulting Group (www.hospitalbillreview.com) a leader in health care fair pricing and medical billing. They have information for every procedure and every hospital and have saved patients $2 million to date. Call (800)906-8085.

Advocacy for Patients www.advocacyforpatients.org) - Patients with a chronic illness can get free information, advice and advocacy services in areas including but not limited to the following:

- How to get your own medical records.
- How to get and keep health insurance.
- How to get health insurance coverage for particular treatments, drugs, and/or therapies.
- How to get private disability insurance coverage.
- How to get Social Security Disability Income. How to assert your rights under the Americans with Disabilities Act.
- How to assert your rights under the Family and Medical Leave Act.
- How to ensure that schools accommodate students with chronic illnesses.

State Mandates

If you have **private** insurance and have been denied coverage for specific medical care or service, check your state mandates at www.cahi.org/cahi_contents/resources/pdf/HealthInsuranceMandates2009.pdf.

Mandates require insurance companies to cover certain health care providers, benefits and patient populations.

Please note: Employer based or group health plans are exempt from state mandates, although they follow separate laws under ERISA. See Chapter one for more information.

Get the Most Out of Your Health Insurance

Check your health plan for additional benefits such as:

- Mail order prescription plans
- Free health screenings and physicals
- Free or discounted gym memberships
- Discounted diet plans (i.e. Weight Watchers, Jenny Craig)
- Free advice from a nurse line

- Cash rewards for healthy living i.e. exercising, weight loss, quitting smoking, stress reduction classes

Shop for Dental Insurance

If you've been to a dentist, you know dental care is expensive. Dental insurance helps but unfortunately, a third of employers do not offer dental insurance, leaving many without dental coverage.

Why is Dental Coverage Important?

The truth is people without dental benefits are 2.5 times more likely NOT to go to the dentist, leading to more dental disease and tooth loss down the road.

One of your options is to shop for a private dental insurance plans but quite honestly, finding a good plan worth the cost can be difficult so you may be better off buying a dental discount plan for about half the cost (see page 118).

When shopping for a dental insurance plan be sure to think about anticipated dental needs for you and your family along with annual premiums (average is $200-$800 a yr. for family of 4), deductibles, co-insurance (amount you're responsible for) and coverage limitations and exclusions.

Search the **National Association of Dental Plans** at http://nadp.org for a directory of dental insurance and discount plan carriers in your state.

AARP and COSTCO also offer their own dental plans through **Delta Dental.** I find their rates competitive with some employer based plans.

- **AARP members** only at http://www3.deltadentalins.com/aarp
- **COSTCO executive members** in CA only http://www.deltadentalins.com/plans_costco

You can also purchase a plan directly through **Delta Dental** at http://www.deltadentalins.com, **which may be cheaper.**

Buy a Dental Discount Plan

Another, more affordable option is a dental discount plan. Even if you are lucky enough to have dental insurance, I'm willing to bet it doesn't provide enough coverage for most of your dental care and includes a deductible and a 20-50% co-insurance (the amount you are responsible for) for most services.

If you do not have dental insurance, you are likely to pay 'retail' prices for your dental care.

What's nice about these discount plans is that **some discount dental plans may be used as a supplement to your dental insurance for additional savings. You will need to check with your dental care provider prior to treatment.**

What about **specialists or orthodontia care** if you or your children need expensive braces?

Most dental insurance plans exclude orthodontia coverage or put a low cap on the amount they will pay. The good news is that many **dental discount plans** will offer discounts from specialist and orthodontists in your area.

In addition, many discount plans offer additional discounts on prescription drugs, eye care, chiropractic care, and hearing devices.

Dental discount plans are NOT insurance plans. Instead, reputable health organizations (Aetna, Cigna, etc.) partner with local dentists and orthodontists who agree to accept a discounted fee from plan members as payment-in-full for services performed.

Check it out... If you're interested in saving money on your dental bills, check out discount plans, membership pricing and dentists in your area at **DentalPlans.Com** (www.dentalplans.com).

For a limited time, Dental Plans. Com is offering readers an additional 10% off all dental discount plans, which includes 3 additional months FREE! Use Coupon Code CUTCOSTSNOW.*

Stay Healthy

This may be a "no brainer" but remember, private health plans are underwritten based on your age, weight, smoking status and past and present health history so **if your insurance company considers you "unhealthy" they can raise your insurance premiums and even deny you coverage.** In Colorado and other states, health insurance companies can and do deny residents coverage if they believe they are unhealthy.

In addition, a recent survey found that employers are ready to push

---

*"*Cut Your Health Care Costs Now!* is an independent contractor for Dentalplans.com, Inc., and is providing internet affiliate services to the company via the internet for which they may earn financial compensation from Dentalplans.com, Inc.

more of the rising costs of health insurance onto their employees in 2010, while expecting them to take more responsibility for managing their health.

The bottom-line... If you do not take care of your health, it could cost YOU more!

Quit Smoking – Read this guide for successfully quitting. http://www.smokefree.gov/pubs/Clearing-The-Air_acc.pdf

FREE Professional MP3 Audio Hypnosis for Smoking Cessation

http://www.freewebs.com/psych11/smoking.htm

Buy Long-Term Care Insurance

Prepare before it's too late. Long-term health care is usually not covered by health insurance. Consider the **average cost of a nursing home is $55,000 a year**.

If you can afford it, long-term care insurance is something everyone should have for many reasons:

- If you want to stay in your own home if you become ill.

- If you do not want to be a burden to your children or other family.
- If you do not have money saved for elder care or a nursing home.

Buying long-term care insurance will help protect you in the event you are unable to care for yourself because of a disability, chronic illness, or mental impairment including:

- Elder frailty
- Parkinson's Disease
- Alzheimer's
- Stroke
- Cerebral palsy
- Multiple sclerosis
- Auto accident

Visit www.naic.org to learn more.

Most **Federal and U.S. Postal Service employees and annuitants, active and retired members of the uniformed services, and their qualified relatives** are eligible for long-term health care coverage under the Federal Long Term Care Insurance Program (FLTCIP).

For eligibility and plan details, contact Long Term Care Partners at (800)582-3337 or www.ltcfeds.com.

Recommended Reading *Your Medical Bills: A Consumer's Guide to Coping with Medical Debt* at http://www.familiesusa.org.

Chapter Five

Pay Less for Prescription Drugs

Do you need help paying for your prescription drugs?

Are you among the increasing number of Americans who are going without their prescription drugs because of increasing drug prices and decreasing health insurance coverage?

Not sure how or where to look for help?

Here are my top suggestions for paying less for prescription drugs:

Check Your Plan's Formulary before You Sign

You can find most insurance company's formularies online. Use the **formula finder** to see if your pills are covered under Medicare plans at http://drugmanager.medicare.gov.

Ask your Pharmacist for a Discount

Did you know most major retail pharmacies have discount programs for the uninsured or cash paying customers?

Be sure you ask your pharmacist about any discounts you may qualify for.

Shop Around

The internet has made it easier to compare prescription drug prices. Search and compare prices at:

- http://www.pharmacychecker.com/
- http://www.destinationrx.com/
- http://www.pillbot.com/
- http://www.medtipster.com/ find prescription drugs and prices available on discount generic programs in pharmacies across the country.

Buyers Beware, some websites that sell medicine:

- Aren't U.S. state-licensed pharmacies or aren't pharmacies at all.
- May give a diagnosis that is not correct and sell medicine that is not right for you or your condition.
- Won't protect your personal information.

Some medication sold online:

- Are fake (counterfeit or "copycat" medicines)
- Are too strong or too weak

- Have dangerous ingredients

- Have expired (are out-of-date)

- Aren't FDA-approved (haven't been checked for safety and effectiveness)

- Aren't made using safe standards

- Aren't safe to use with other medicine or products you use

- Aren't labeled, stored, or shipped correctly

The FDA says that you should only buy online prescription drugs from a pharmacy if it:

1. **Is located in the United States and licensed by the state board of pharmacy where the Web site is operating.** Check www.nabp.net for a list of state boards of pharmacy.

2. **Has a licensed pharmacist to answer your questions.**

3. **Requires a prescription** from your doctor or other health care professional who is licensed in the United States to write prescriptions for medicine.

4. **Has a way for you to talk to a person** if you have problems.

Use Mail Order

Getting your prescriptions through the mail can save you a lot of time and money. For example, you may be able to get a 3-month supply of your medication for the cost of 1 month's supply.

Most group and private insurance plans have partnered with pharmacy benefit managers (PBM) such as Caremark, Medco, and Express Scripts. Check your insurance policy for information.

Ask for Cheaper Brand Drug Equivalents

Insurance companies are getting pickier about the drugs they cover. You may have noticed you have to pay more out of pocket for some drugs vs. others and this varies from plan to plan. Many plans have different pricing lists for more expensive drugs.

To offset the additional costs to you, ask your provider to prescribe a less expensive drug equivalent. For example, there are many brand name drugs that treat acid reflux and research shows very little if any difference among them besides prices.

A word of caution: It is perfectly legal for pharmacists to switchprescription drugs without your knowledge so be sure it is your physician doing the switching and NOT your pharmacist.

Go Generic

According the Generic Pharmaceutical Association, generic drugs have saved Americans $734 billion dollars over the last 10 years. Some retail chains offer popular generics for just $4 for a 30-day supply. Talk to your health care provider to see if switching your particular medication to generic is best for you.

Generic Drug Discount Programs

CVS/pharmacy Health Savings Pass (www.cvs.com)

WalMart Generics Program Drug List (www.walmart.com)

K-Mart Generics Program Drug List (www.rxassist.org/providers/documents/90DayGenericsFormulary SheetJuly2007_000.pdf)

Target Generics Program Drug List (http://sites.target.com/site/en/health/generic_drugs.jsp).

Rx Outreach (www.rxoutreach.com) 800-769-3880 - They claim to have the lowest possible prices for over 400 generic drugs for individuals and families with incomes of up to 300 percent of the federal poverty level. For a family of four, this amount is about $63,600 per year. People may take advantage of the program even if they receive medicine through another discount program.

Xubex (www.xubex.com) (866) 699-8239 - offers low cost and **FREE medications** for virtually all brand or generic medications.

Discount Pharmacies

Costco (www.costco.com) and Sam's club (www.samsclub.com) pharmacies often have competitive prices. **Membership is not required to use the pharmacy services.** Costco has a mail order pharmacy service, with no additional charges for standard shipping.

Are You a Veteran or a Dependent of a Veteran?

Veterans, retired military personnel, and their dependents may be eligible for prescription drug assistance or coverage from the Department of Veterans Affairs' Health Administration.

Call 877-222-8387 or visit **TRICARE**, the U.S. Department of Defense Military Health System at www.tricare.osd.mil.

Pharmaceutical & Other Prescription Assistance Programs

Having at least one chronic condition more than doubles the likelihood of reporting unmet prescription drug needs. The good news is that there are many drug assistance programs that can help.

- **www.needymeds.com**
  A nonprofit organization offering a searchable database of patient assistance programs offered by drug manufacturers and others. Application forms provided.

- **www.xubex.com** (866) 699-8239 - Offers low cost and **FREE medications** for virtually all Rx brand and generic medications for those who qualify.

- **www.rarediseases.org**
  A website of the **National Organization for Rare Disorders** (NORD) provides a list of medication assistance programs for uninsured or underinsured people with specific rare conditions, including multiple sclerosis (MS).

- **www.helpingpatients.org**
  The **Pharmaceutical Research and Manufacturers of America**

- (PhRMA) lists all the patient assistance programs of its members, and helps users determine their eligibility online.

- **www.pparx.org Partnership for Prescription Assistance** brings together America's pharmaceutical companies, doctors, other health care providers, patient advocacy organizations and community groups to help qualifying patients without prescription drug coverage get free or low-cost medicines through the public or private program that's right for them.

- **www.themedicineprogram.com** Helps people obtain free prescription drugs for patients in need through various patient assistance programs.

- **www.rxhope.com** The largest independent web-based patient assistance resource. Search for prescription drug help from a comprehensive list of current Patient Assistance Programs.

- **www.benefitscheckup.org** For people 55 years and older. Provides a confidential, personalized report of public and private prescription drug assistance programs.

State Assistance Programs

Some states have created a plan to launch some type of program to provide pharmaceutical coverage or assistance, primarily to low-income elderly and/or people with disabilities who do not qualify for Medicaid. The programs offer savings paid for by the state's government.

Two organizations list details of each state's program:

The **Medicare Rights Center** - go to www.medicarerights.org *Medicare Basics, Help Paying for Prescription Drugs*

The National Conference of State Legislatures www.ncsl.org/programs/health/drugaid.htm. Offers a no-cost online registration.

Discount Drug Cards & Coupons

Discount cards rely on the large volume purchasing power of the state to negotiate considerable discounts on brand and generic drugs. There are many types of drug discount cards. Some provide big savings, others do not. It may best to use certain discount cards with certain drugs.

BIG TIP: Some companies only offer discounts to those without insurance or without prescription drug coverage. If you have prescription drug coverage but have reached your limit, I highly recommend you attach a letter from your insurance company to your application.

Here are my top picks:

> **NeedyMeds Discount Card** (www.needymeds.org/indices/discountcards.shtml) provides **a 20-60% discount** on many medicines.

> **Save** BIG by searching for *drug coupons, discount co-pay and savings cards and FREE 30 day trials* for popular brand name drugs such as Nexium, Prevacid, Crestor, Lipitor and more at www.needymeds.org/indices/coupon.shtml.

> Print your **FREE Prescription Drug Card** at http://freedrugcard.us and receive **savings of up to 75%** at more than 54,000 national and regional pharmacies.

> **Together RxAccess** (www.togetherrxaccess.com) For people without insurance. This drug discount card is

sponsored by 10 major pharmaceutical companies--Abbott Laboratories, AstraZeneca, Bristol Meyers Squibb, Glaxo Smith Kline, Johnson & Johnson, Novartis, Pfizer, Sanofi Aventis, Takeda and TAP Pharmaceuticals. The card is free and offers **a 25%-40%* discount** on over 300 brand-name and generic prescription drugs as well as other prescription products, such as glucose test strips.

Other Discount Websites

FamiliesUSA (www.familiesusa.org) provides information on new Medicare drug information.

$25 Dollar Prescription Eyeglasses (http://25dollareyeglasses.net)
Diabetic Savings Plan (www.diabeticsavingsplan.com)

Conclusion

So there you have it. I have given you all the information and "insider" tips you need to help cut your health care costs today!

I hope you have found this to be a valuable resource and that you will soon be on your way to saving BIG on your health care.

I welcome your feedback at www.lowerhealthcarebills.com.

Wishing you optimum health,

Brandi Funk, FNP

Notes